AUTOIMMUNE PALEO DIET COOKBOOK

Nourishing Meals to Restore Balance and Wellness

Myke Sez

TABLE OF CONTENTS

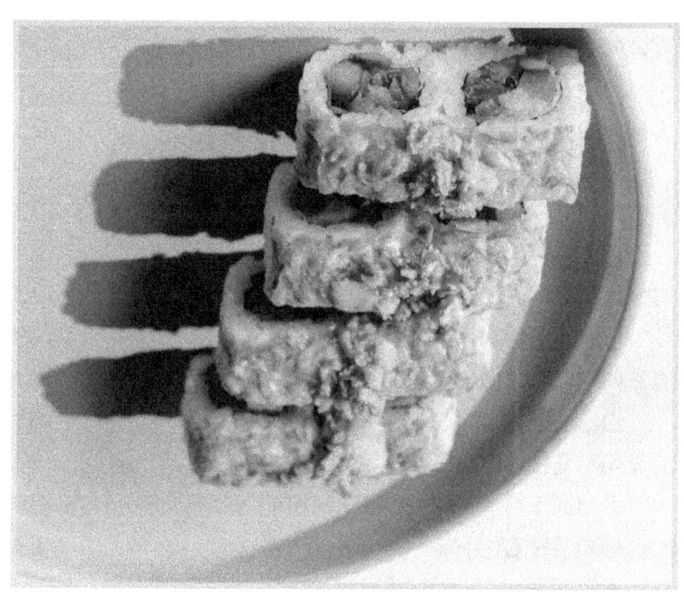

INTRODUCTION

Welcome to the 'Autoimmune Paleo Diet Cookbook,' a labor of love that demonstrates the transformational power of food. If you've picked up this book, chances are you or someone you care about is grappling with an autoimmune condition. Either you are newly diagnosed, an experienced fighter, or simply want to support your health in the best way possible, this cookbook is for you.

I started this journey much like many of you—confused, frustrated, and overwhelmed by the myriad of information available. My own experience with autoimmune disease led me down countless paths, each promising relief but often leading to more questions than answers. It was through this maze of uncertainty that I discovered the Autoimmune Paleo (AIP) Diet, a beacon of hope that finally offered tangible results.

The AIP Diet isn't just another trend; it's a scientifically backed approach that focuses on repairing the gut, reducing inflammation, and providing your body with the nutrients it needs to thrive. It's about stripping away the common triggers that exacerbate autoimmune symptoms and embracing a diet that nourishes you from the inside out.

But let's be real—changing your diet is no small feat. It can be daunting to give up foods that have been staples in your life for years. You might be wondering how you'll manage without your morning toast or your favorite pasta dish. Trust me, I've been there. The key is to shift your mindset from one of deprivation to one of abundance. Instead of focusing on what you can't have, let's celebrate the vibrant, delicious, and health-boosting foods you can enjoy.

This cookbook is here to guide you through that transition with recipes that are not only compliant with the AIP guidelines but also flavorful, satisfying, and easy to prepare. You'll find everything from hearty breakfasts to soul-soothing soups, from vibrant salads to comforting main courses, and of course, treats that will make you forget you're even on a diet.

Each recipe has been meticulously crafted with the intention of making your life easier and your meals more enjoyable. I've included tips on meal prepping, substitutions for common allergens, and ways to adapt recipes to suit your individual needs. You'll also find personal anecdotes and insights that I hope will resonate with you, offering encouragement and a sense of connection.

Food is more than just sustenance; it's a source of joy, connection, and healing. As you look through the recipes on these pages, I invite you to approach the process with an open heart and a curious palette. Cooking can be therapeutic, allowing you to reconnect with your body and its impulses. It's an opportunity to create a new narrative about food, one that empowers you to take charge of your health and well-being.

Remember, this is not a sprint but a marathon. There will be days when you slip up, and that's okay. Be gentle to yourself and appreciate your minor accomplishments along the way. The journey to wellness is unique for each of us, and there is no one-size-fits-all approach. Listen to your body, trust the process, and know that you are not alone

CHAPTER ONE

GETTING STARTED WITH AUTOIMMUNE PALEO DIET

Getting started on the Autoimmune Paleo (AIP) journey can feel overwhelming, but understanding the basics and having a solid plan can make the transition smoother and more manageable. This section will guide you through the essentials of getting started with the AIP diet, from understanding autoimmune diseases to meal planning and preparation.

Understanding Autoimmune Diseases

Autoimmune diseases occur when the immune system, which is designed to protect the body from harmful invaders, mistakenly attacks healthy cells.This can cause a variety of symptoms, depending on whatever area of the body is afflicted. Common autoimmune diseases include rheumatoid arthritis, lupus, multiple sclerosis, and Hashimoto's thyroiditis, among many others.

While the exact cause of autoimmune diseases is still unknown, it is believed that a combination of genetic, environmental, and lifestyle factors contribute to their development. Diet plays a significant role in managing these conditions because certain foods can trigger inflammation and exacerbate symptoms. This is where the AIP diet comes into play.

What is the Autoimmune Paleo Diet?

The Autoimmune Paleo Diet, often referred to as AIP, is a specialized elimination diet designed to reduce inflammation, repair the gut, and help identify food sensitivities that may trigger autoimmune responses. The AIP diet takes the basic principles of the Paleo diet (which focuses on whole, unprocessed foods) a step further by eliminating additional foods that can potentially irritate the gut and contribute to inflammation.

The Science Behind AIP

The AIP diet is grounded in the idea that our modern diet, rich in processed foods, sugar, and artificial additives, can damage the gut lining, leading to a condition known as "leaky gut." When the gut is compromised, undigested food particles and toxins can leak into the bloodstream, triggering an immune response. By removing foods that are known to be problematic and focusing on nutrient-dense, anti-inflammatory foods, the AIP diet aims to repair the gut, reduce systemic inflammation, and, as a result, alleviate autoimmune symptoms.

Benefits of AIP

The benefits of following the AIP diet can be significant for those with autoimmune conditions:

Reduced Inflammation: By eliminating inflammatory foods, the body can start to repair and reduce chronic inflammation.

Improved Gut Health: AIP focuses on gut-repairing foods like bone broth and fermented vegetables, which can help restore the gut lining.

Symptom Relief: Many people experience a reduction in autoimmune symptoms such as fatigue, joint pain, and digestive issues.

Increased Nutrient Intake: The diet emphasizes nutrient-dense foods, ensuring your body gets the vitamins and minerals it needs.

Better Food Awareness: Through the elimination phase and subsequent reintroductions, you'll learn which foods your body tolerates well and which ones to avoid.

Foods to Avoid on AIP

The AIP diet eliminates foods that are known to trigger inflammation and immune responses. Here is a complete list of foods to avoid:

Grains: Wheat, rice, corn, oats, barley, quinoa, etc.

Legumes: Beans, lentils, soy, peanuts, etc.

Dairy: Milk, cheese, yogurt, butter, etc.

Nuts and Seeds: Almonds, cashews, chia seeds, sunflower seeds, etc.

Nightshade Vegetables: Tomatoes, potatoes, eggplants, peppers, etc.

Processed Foods: Any food with artificial additives, preservatives, or refined sugars.

Eggs: All types of eggs, as they can be inflammatory for some people.

Alcohol and Caffeine: Both can disrupt gut health and trigger immune responses.

Foods to Include on AIP

While the list of foods to avoid might seem extensive, there are plenty of delicious and nutritious foods you can enjoy on the AIP diet:

Vegetables: Leafy greens, carrots, broccoli, cauliflower, zucchini, etc.

Fruits: Apples, berries, bananas, pears, etc.

Meat and Fish: Grass-fed beef, poultry, wild-caught fish, lamb, etc.

Healthy fats: Olive oil, coconut oil, and avocado oil.

Herbs and Spices: Basil, oregano, turmeric, ginger, etc. (excluding seed-based spices)

Bone Broth: Rich in collagen and gut-healing properties.

Fermented Foods: Sauerkraut, kimchi, kombucha, etc., which support gut health.

Tips for Transitioning to AIP

Transitioning to the AIP diet can be challenging, but these tips can help make the process smoother:

Educate Yourself: Understand the principles of the AIP diet and why certain foods are eliminated.

Start Slowly: Gradually eliminate foods from your diet rather than all at once to make the transition easier.

Plan Your Meals: Having a meal plan in place can prevent last-minute food choices that might not be AIP-compliant.

Batch Cook: Prepare meals in advance to save time and ensure you always have AIP-friendly options available.

Find Support: Join AIP communities, whether online or in person, to share experiences and get support.

Listen to your body. Pay attention to how your body reacts to different meals and change your diet accordingly.

Meal Planning and Preparation

Effective meal planning and preparation are key to success on the AIP diet. Below are some strategies to help you stay on track:

Weekly Planning: Set aside time each week to plan your meals and make a shopping list.

Grocery Shopping: Buy fresh, whole foods and avoid the processed food aisles.

Batch Cooking: Cook large quantities of meals that can be stored in the refrigerator or freezer for later use.

Prep Ingredients: Wash and chop vegetables, marinate meats, and prepare snacks ahead of time.

Stay Organized: Keep your kitchen organized with AIP-friendly ingredients and tools for easy meal preparation.

Use Leftovers: Include leftovers in your meal plan to reduce waste and save time.

By understanding autoimmune diseases, knowing which foods to avoid and include, and following these tips for transitioning and meal planning, you'll be well-equipped to start your AIP journey with confidence and ease. Remember, the goal is to support your body's healing process and improve your overall well-being.

CHAPTER TWO

BREAKFAST RECIPES

Starting your day with a nutritious and delicious breakfast is key to maintaining energy and supporting your health, especially on the Autoimmune Paleo (AIP) diet. Here are some creative and satisfying breakfast recipes that adhere to AIP guidelines.

01. <u>AIP Smoothie Bowls</u>

Smoothie bowls are a fun and versatile way to pack a lot of nutrients into your breakfast. You can pair up ingredients according to what you have readily available.

<u>Ingredients:</u>

1 cup frozen berries (blueberries, strawberries, raspberries)

1 frozen banana

1/2 cup coconut milk or other AIP-compliant milk

1 tablespoon coconut oil

1 tablespoon collagen peptides (optional)

Fresh fruit, coconut flakes, and AIP granola for toppings

Instructions:

- ❖ In a blender, combine the frozen berries, frozen banana, coconut milk, and coconut oil.
- ❖ Combine until smooth and creamy, adding additional coconut milk as needed to reach the texture you want.
- ❖ Pour the smoothie into a bowl and top with fresh fruit, coconut flakes, and AIP granola.
- ❖ Enjoy immediately for a refreshing and energizing breakfast.

02. Grain-Free Pancakes

These grain-free pancakes are fluffy, delicious, and perfect for a leisurely weekend breakfast or brunch.

Ingredients:

1/2 cup cassava flour

1/4 cup coconut flour

1/2 teaspoon baking soda

Pinch of sea salt

1/2 cup coconut milk

1/4 cup water

2 tablespoons coconut oil, melted

1 tablespoon honey (optional)

1 teaspoon apple cider vinegar

Instructions:

- ❖ In a mixing bowl, whisk together the cassava flour, coconut flour, baking soda, and salt.
- ❖ In a separate bowl, mix the coconut milk, water, melted coconut oil, honey, and apple cider vinegar.
- ❖ Pour the wet ingredients into the dry ingredients and whisk until thoroughly blended.
- ❖ Heat a skillet over medium heat and lightly coat it with coconut oil.

- ❖ Pour 1/4 cup batter into the heated skillet for each pancake. Cook for 2-3 minutes per side, or until golden brown.
- ❖ Serve with fresh fruit, coconut yogurt, or a drizzle of maple syrup (if tolerated).

03. <u>Sweet Potato Hash with Greens</u>

This hearty sweet potato hash is packed with nutrients and flavor, making it a perfect way to start your day.

<u>Ingredients:</u>

2 medium sweet potatoes, peeled and diced

1 tablespoon coconut oil

1 small onion, diced

2 cloves garlic, minced

1 cup chopped kale or spinach

Sea salt and black pepper (omit if sensitive to pepper) to taste

Fresh herbs (parsley, cilantro) for garnish

Instructions:

- ❖ In a big pan, heat the coconut oil over medium heat.
- ❖ Add the diced sweet potatoes and cook for about 10 minutes, stirring occasionally, until they begin to soften.
- ❖ Add the diced onion and garlic to the skillet and cook for another 5 minutes, until the onions are translucent and the sweet potatoes are tender.
- ❖ Stir in the chopped kale or spinach and cook for an additional 2-3 minutes, until wilted.
- ❖ Garnish with sea salt as desired.
- ❖ Garnish with fresh herbs and serve immediately.

04. Coconut Yogurt Parfait

This simple yet elegant coconut yogurt parfait is a delightful way to enjoy a dairy-free, gut-friendly breakfast.

Ingredients:

1 cup coconut yogurt (store-bought or homemade)

Fresh fruit (berries, sliced kiwi, banana)

AIP granola

Unsweetened coconut flakes

A drizzle of honey (optional)

Instructions:

- ❖ In a serving glass or bowl, layer the coconut yogurt, fresh fruit, and AIP granola.
- ❖ Continue the steps until you've used all of the ingredients.
- ❖ Top with unsweetened coconut flakes and a drizzle of honey, if desired.
- ❖ Serve immediately and enjoy the refreshing, creamy flavors.

05. Egg-Free Breakfast Muffins

These egg-free breakfast muffins are perfect for those busy mornings when you need a quick, grab-and-go option.

Ingredients:

1 cup grated zucchini

1/2 cup grated carrot

1/4 cup coconut flour

1/4 cup cassava flour

1/2 teaspoon baking soda

1/4 teaspoon sea salt

1/4 cup coconut oil, melted

1/4 cup unsweetened applesauce

1 tablespoon apple cider vinegar

1 tablespoon honey (optional)

Instructions:

- ❖ Heat the oven to 350°F/175°C and line a muffin tray with paper liners.

- ❖ In a large mixing bowl, combine the grated zucchini, grated carrot, coconut flour, cassava flour, baking soda, and sea salt.

- ❖ In a separate bowl, mix the melted coconut oil, applesauce, apple cider vinegar, and honey.

- ❖ Pour the wet ingredients into the dry ingredients and whisk until thoroughly blended.

- ❖ Distribute the batter equally into the muffin cups.
- ❖ Bake for 20 to 25 minutes, or until a knife poked in the middle comes out clean.
- ❖ Leave the muffins to cool down in their tins for a few minutes before moving to a wire structure to finish cooling.
- ❖ Enjoy as a quick breakfast or snack throughout the week.

These recipes are designed to make your mornings easier and more enjoyable while adhering to the AIP guidelines. With a bit of planning and creativity, you can enjoy a variety of delicious and satisfying breakfasts that support your health and well-being.

CHAPTER THREE

LUNCH RECIPES

Lunchtime can be a delightful and nourishing part of your day, especially with these AIP-friendly recipes. These dishes are not only compliant with the AIP diet but also delicious and easy to prepare. Let's explore some mouth-watering lunch options;

01. Zucchini Noodles with Pesto

Zucchini noodles, or "zoodles," are a fantastic alternative to traditional pasta. Paired with a vibrant, homemade pesto, this dish is light, flavorful, and perfect for a satisfying lunch.

Ingredients:

2 medium zucchinis, spiralized into noodles

1 cup fresh basil leaves

1/4 cup olive oil

1/4 cup pumpkin seeds (optional)

1 clove garlic

Juice of 1 lemon

Sea salt to taste

Cherry tomatoes (optional) for garnish

Instructions:

- ❖ Make the Pesto: In a food processor, combine basil leaves, olive oil, pumpkin seeds (if using), garlic, lemon juice, and sea salt. Blend until smooth.
- ❖ Prepare the Zoodles: In a large pan, lightly sauté the zucchini noodles for 2-3 minutes, until just tender but still firm.
- ❖ Combine: Toss the warm zoodles with the pesto until evenly coated.
- ❖ Serve: Garnish with cherry tomatoes if desired. Serve immediately and enjoy the fresh, herby flavors.

02. Chicken and Avocado Salad

This chicken and avocado salad is a protein-packed, nutrient-dense meal that's both creamy and satisfying. It's quick to prepare and perfect for a healthy lunch.

Ingredients:

2 cooked chicken breasts, shredded

1 ripe avocado, diced

1/2 red onion, finely chopped

1 cucumber, diced

1 cup cherry tomatoes, halved

Juice of 1 lime

2 tablespoons olive oil

Fresh cilantro or parsley, chopped

Sea salt and black pepper to taste (omit pepper if sensitive)

Instructions:

- ❖ Combine Ingredients: In a large bowl, combine the shredded chicken, diced avocado, chopped red onion, cucumber, and cherry tomatoes.
- ❖ Dress the Salad: In a small bowl, whisk together the lime juice, olive oil, and sea

salt. Sprinkle over the salad and gently stir to mix.

- ❖ Garnish and Serve: Sprinkle with fresh cilantro or parsley. Serve immediately or chill in the fridge for a refreshing cold salad.

03. <u>Sweet Potato and Kale Soup</u>

This comforting soup is perfect for a cozy lunch. Packed with nutrients and flavor, it's a great way to stay warm and full.

<u>Ingredients:</u>

2 large sweet potatoes, peeled and cubed

1 onion, chopped

2 cloves garlic, minced

4 cups chicken or vegetable broth (AIP-compliant)

2 cups chopped kale

1 tablespoon coconut oil

1 teaspoon turmeric

Sea salt and black pepper to taste (omit pepper if sensitive)

Fresh herbs for garnish

Instructions:

- ❖ Sauté Vegetables: In a large pot, heat the coconut oil over medium heat. Sauté the onions and garlic until fragrant and transparent.

- ❖ Add Sweet Potatoes: Add the cubed sweet potatoes and turmeric, stirring to coat. Add the stock and bring to a boil.

- ❖ Simmer: Reduce heat and let the soup simmer for about 20 minutes, until the sweet potatoes are tender.

- ❖ Add Kale: Stir in the chopped kale and cook for an additional 5 minutes.

- ❖ Puree (Optional): To achieve a creamier texture, use an immersion blender to partially puree the soup.

- ❖ Season and Serve: Season with sea salt and black pepper to taste. Serve hot, garnished with fresh herbs.

04. <u>Tuna-Stuffed Avocados</u>

This simple yet delicious dish combines the creamy texture of avocado with a flavorful tuna salad. It's quick to prepare and perfect for a light yet filling lunch.

<u>Ingredients:</u>

2 ripe avocados, halved and pitted

1 can of tuna in water, drained

2 tablespoons coconut yogurt or AIP-compliant mayo

1 celery stalk, finely chopped

1 tablespoon fresh lemon juice

Sea salt to taste

Fresh dill or parsley for garnish

<u>Instructions:</u>

- ❖ Prepare Tuna Salad: In a bowl, mix the drained tuna with coconut yogurt or mayo, chopped celery, lemon juice, and sea salt.
- ❖ Stuff Avocados: Spoon the tuna mixture into the avocado halves.

❖ Garnish and Serve: Sprinkle with fresh dill or parsley. Serve immediately and enjoy the combination of creamy and savory flavors.

05. <u>Collard Wraps with Turkey and Veggies</u>

These collard wraps are a fresh and fun way to enjoy a sandwich without the bread. Packed with lean turkey and crunchy vegetables, they make a healthy and satisfying lunch.

<u>Ingredients:</u>

4 large collard green leaves

8 slices of cooked turkey breast

1 red bell pepper, thinly sliced

1 cucumber, julienned

1 carrot, julienned

1 avocado, sliced

2 tablespoons coconut aminos (optional for extra flavor)

Sea salt and black pepper to taste (omit pepper if sensitive)

<u>Instructions:</u>

- ❖ Prepare Collard Leaves: Rinse the collard leaves and pat dry. Carefully cut off the thick stem at the bottom of each leaf.
- ❖ Assemble Wraps: Lay a collard leaf flat and place 2 slices of turkey breast in the center. Top with slices of red bell pepper, cucumber, carrot, and avocado.
- ❖ Season: Drizzle with coconut aminos if using and season with sea salt.
- ❖ Wrap: Fold the sides of the collard leaf over the fillings and then roll up tightly from the bottom, like a burrito.
- ❖ Serving: If desired, cut in half and serve instantly. Enjoy the fresh, crunchy textures and vibrant flavors.

These AIP-friendly lunch recipes are not only delicious but also packed with nutrients to keep you energized throughout the day. With a bit of preparation, you can enjoy a variety of meals that support your health and delight your taste buds.

CHAPTER FOUR

DINNER RECIPES

Dinnertime is an opportunity to wind down, nourish your body, and enjoy a wholesome meal. Here are some delectable AIP-friendly dinner recipes that are not only healthy but also packed with flavor. These recipes are designed to be satisfying and supportive of your health goals on the AIP diet.

01. <u>Herb-Roasted Chicken with Vegetables</u>

A classic roast chicken is elevated with a medley of herbs and paired with a variety of roasted vegetables. This dish is comforting, hearty, and perfect for a family dinner.

<u>Ingredients:</u>

1 whole chicken (about 4-5 pounds)

1/4 cup olive oil

2 tablespoons fresh rosemary, chopped

2 tablespoons fresh thyme, chopped

4 garlic cloves, minced

Juice of 1 lemon

Sea salt and black pepper to taste (omit pepper if sensitive)

4 carrots, peeled and cut into chunks

4 parsnips, peeled and cut into chunks

1 large onion, cut into wedges

2 cups Brussels sprouts, halved

Instructions:

- ❖ Heat the oven to 375°F (190°C)

- ❖ Prepare Chicken: Rinse the chicken inside and out, and pat dry with paper towels. Place it in a roasting pan.

- ❖ Make Herb Mixture: In a small bowl, combine the olive oil, chopped rosemary, thyme, minced garlic, lemon juice, sea salt, and black pepper. Rub this mixture all over the chicken, making sure to get under the skin and inside the cavity.

- ❖ Prepare Vegetables: Arrange the carrots, parsnips, onion wedges, and Brussels sprouts around the chicken in the roasting pan. Sprinkle with olive oil and sprinkle with sea salt.

- ❖ Roast: Roast the chicken for about 1.5 to 2 hours, or until the internal temperature reaches 165°F (75°C) and the juices run clear. Rub the chicken with the pan juices halfway through the cooking process.
- ❖ Rest and Serve: Let the chicken rest for 10 minutes before carving. Serve with the roasted vegetables.

02. <u>Baked Salmon with Lemon and Dill</u>

This baked salmon recipe is simple yet bursting with fresh flavors. The combination of lemon and dill enhances the natural taste of the salmon, making it a light and healthy dinner option.

<u>Ingredients:</u>

4 salmon fillets

2 tablespoons olive oil

Juice of 1 lemon

2 tablespoons fresh dill, chopped

1 garlic clove, minced

Sea salt to taste

Lemon slices for garnish

Instructions:

- ❖ Preheat the oven to 400 degrees Fahrenheit (200 degrees Celsius).
- ❖ Prepare Marinade: In a small bowl, mix the olive oil, lemon juice, chopped dill, minced garlic, and sea salt.
- ❖ Marinate Salmon: Put the salmon fillets on a baking sheet lined with parchment paper. Brush the marinade over the fillets, making sure they are well coated.
- ❖ Bake: Bake the salmon for 12-15 minutes, or until the fish flakes easily with a fork.
- ❖ Serve: Garnish with lemon slices and extra dill if desired. Serve immediately with your favorite AIP-friendly side dishes.

03. <u>Beef and Broccoli Stir-Fry</u>

This beef and broccoli stir-fry is a quick and delicious dinner that's packed with protein and veggies. The savory sauce ties everything together for a satisfying meal.

<u>Ingredients:</u>

1 pound beef sirloin, thinly sliced

2 tablespoons coconut aminos

1 tablespoon apple cider vinegar

2 tablespoons olive oil

4 cups broccoli florets

1 red bell pepper, sliced

3 cloves garlic, minced

1 tablespoon fresh ginger, grated

Sea salt to taste

<u>Instructions:</u>

- ❖ Marinate Beef: In a bowl, combine the sliced beef, coconut aminos, and apple cider vinegar.Allow to marinade for at least 15 minutes.
- ❖ Cook Beef: Heat 1 tablespoon of olive oil in a large skillet or wok over medium-high

heat. Stir-fry the marinated beef for 5-7 minutes, or until it is browned and thoroughly cooked. Remove the steak from the skillet and set it aside.

❖ Cook Vegetables: In the same skillet, heat the remaining olive oil. Combine broccoli, red bell pepper, garlic, and ginger. Stir-fry for approximately 5 minutes, or until the vegetables are soft but still crunchy.

❖ Combine and Serve: Return the beef to the skillet and toss to combine with the vegetables. Season with sea salt to taste. Serve hot over cauliflower rice or by itself.

04. <u>Lamb Meatballs with Mint Sauce</u>

These lamb meatballs are packed with flavor and paired with a refreshing mint sauce. They make for a hearty and flavorful dinner that's sure to impress.

<u>Ingredients for Meatballs:</u>

1 pound ground lamb

1/4 cup finely chopped onion

2 garlic cloves, minced

1 tablespoon fresh mint, chopped

1 tablespoon fresh parsley, chopped

1 teaspoon sea salt

1/2 teaspoon ground cinnamon

<u>Ingredients for Mint Sauce:</u>

1/2 cup coconut yogurt

2 tablespoons fresh mint, chopped

1 tablespoon fresh lemon juice

Sea salt to taste

<u>Instructions:</u>

- ❖ Preheat the oven to 400 degrees Fahrenheit (200 degrees Celsius).
- ❖ Make Meatballs: In a large bowl, combine the ground lamb, chopped onion, minced garlic, mint, parsley, sea salt, and cinnamon. Mix thoroughly until all components are evenly combined. Form the mixture into small meatballs approximately an inch in diameter.

- ❖ Bake Meatballs: Put the meatballs on a baking sheet lined with parchment paper. Bake the meatballs for 15-20 minutes, or until thoroughly done.
- ❖ Prepare Mint Sauce: While the meatballs are baking, make the mint sauce. In a small bowl, mix the coconut yogurt, chopped mint, lemon juice, and sea salt.
- ❖ Serve: Serve the meatballs with the mint sauce on the side.Complement with roasted veggies or a fresh salad.

05. <u>Cauliflower Rice Sushi Rolls</u>

These cauliflower rice sushi rolls are a fun and creative way to enjoy sushi without the grains. They are light, fresh, and can be customized with your favorite AIP-friendly fillings.

<u>Ingredients:</u>

1 small head of cauliflower, riced

1 tablespoon coconut oil

4-6 nori sheets

AIP-friendly fillings (such as cucumber, avocado, cooked shrimp, and carrots)

Coconut aminos for dipping

Instructions:

- ❖ Prepare Cauliflower Rice: In a large skillet, heat the coconut oil over medium heat. Add the riced cauliflower and cook for about 5-7 minutes, until soft and tender. Allow to cool slightly.

- ❖ Assemble Sushi Rolls: Place a nori sheet on a bamboo sushi mat or a piece of parchment paper. Spread a thin layer of cauliflower rice over the nori, leaving about an inch at the top edge.

- ❖ Fillings: Set up your desired fillings in a line along the bottom border of the rice.

- ❖ Roll: Carefully roll the nori sheet, using the mat or parchment paper to help. To seal the roll, wet the nori's top edge with a little water.

❖ Slice and Serve: Slice the sushi roll into bite-sized pieces using a sharp knife. Serve with coconut aminos for dipping.

These AIP-friendly dinner recipes offer a variety of flavors and textures to keep your meals exciting and nutritious. With a little creativity and preparation, you can enjoy delicious dinners that support your health and well-being.

CHAPTER FIVE

SIDE DISHES AND SNACKS

Finding satisfying side dishes and snacks can be a delightful part of following the Autoimmune Paleo (AIP) diet. These recipes are designed to be both nutritious and flavorful, ensuring you don't feel deprived while staying compliant with AIP guidelines.

01. Roasted Root Vegetables

Roasting brings out the natural sweetness of root vegetables, making them a delicious and nutrient-dense side dish. You can mix and match your favorite root veggies for a colorful and tasty addition to any meal.

Ingredients:

2 big carrots, peeled and cut into bits

2 parsnips, peeled and cut into chunks

1 sweet potato, peeled and cubed

1 beet, peeled and cubed

2 tablespoons olive oil

1 teaspoon sea salt

Fresh herbs (rosemary, thyme) for garnish

Instructions:

- ❖ Preheat the oven to 400 degrees Fahrenheit (200 degrees Celsius).

- ❖ Prepare Vegetables: In a large bowl, combine the carrots, parsnips, sweet potato, and beet. Sprinkle olive oil and season with sea salt. Stir to coat uniformly.

- ❖ Roasted Vegetables: Place the vegetables in a single layer on a baking sheet. Roast the vegetables for 25-30 minutes, or until soft and lightly browned, tossing halfway through.

- ❖ Serve: Garnish with fresh herbs and serve hot.

These roasted root vegetables make a perfect accompaniment to any main course.

02. <u>AIP Guacamole and Plantain Chips</u>

This AIP-friendly guacamole, served with crunchy plantain chips, is an excellent snack or appetizer. It's creamy, crispy, and packed with flavor.

<u>Ingredients for Guacamole:</u>

2 ripe avocados

1 lime, juiced

1/4 cup finely chopped red onion

1 garlic clove, minced

1/4 cup chopped fresh cilantro

Sea salt to taste

<u>Ingredients for Plantain Chips:</u>

2 green plantains

2 tablespoons coconut oil, melted

Sea salt to taste

<u>Instructions:</u>

- ❖ Prepare Guacamole: In a medium bowl, mash the avocados with a fork until smooth. Add the lime juice, red onion, garlic, cilantro, and sea salt. Mix well and set aside.

- ❖ Preheat Oven: Preheat the oven to 375°F (190°C).

- ❖ Make Plantain Chips: Peel the plantains and slice them thinly. In a large bowl, toss the plantain slices with melted coconut oil and sea salt.

- ❖ Bake Plantain Chips: Arrange the plantain slices in a single layer on a baking sheet. Bake for 15-20 minutes, flipping halfway through, until they are golden and crispy.

- ❖ Serve: Serve the guacamole with the plantain chips for dipping. Enjoy this delicious and satisfying snack.

<u>03, Fermented Vegetables</u>

Fermented vegetables are a fantastic way to support gut health while enjoying a tangy and crunchy snack. You can ferment almost any vegetable, but here's a basic recipe to get you started.

<u>Ingredients:</u>

1 small cabbage, shredded

2 carrots, grated

1 tablespoon sea salt

1-2 cups filtered water (if needed)

1-2 tablespoons grated ginger (optional for extra flavor)

Instructions:

* ❖ Prepare Vegetables: In a large bowl, combine the shredded cabbage, grated carrots, and sea salt. Massage the vegetables with your hands for about 5-10 minutes until they start to release their juices.

* ❖ Pack into Jar: Pack the vegetables tightly into a clean glass jar, pressing down firmly so the juices cover the vegetables. If there isn't enough liquid, add a little filtered water to ensure the veggies are submerged.

* ❖ Ferment: Place a cloth over the jar and fasten it with an elastic band. Let it sit at room temperature for 3-7 days, checking daily to ensure the vegetables remain submerged and pressing them down if needed.

- ❖ Taste and Store: Taste the fermented vegetables after a few days. When they reach your desired level of tanginess, transfer the jar to the refrigerator. Excellent as a side dish or snack.

04. Butternut Squash Fries

These butternut squash fries are a delicious and healthy alternative to regular fries. They are crunchy, somewhat sweet, and ideal for dipping

Ingredients:

One large butternut squash, peeled and sliced into fries

2 tablespoons olive oil

1 teaspoon sea salt

1/2 teaspoon ground cinnamon (optional)

Instructions:

- ❖ Preheat the oven to 425°F (220°C).
- ❖ Prepare Squash: In a large bowl, toss the butternut squash fries with olive oil, sea salt, and ground cinnamon if using.

- ❖ Bake Fries: Arrange the fries in a single layer on a baking pan. Bake for 25-30 minutes, flipping halfway through, until the fries are golden and crispy.
- ❖ Serve: Serve immediately with your favorite AIP-friendly dipping sauce. These fries are ideal as a side dish or snack.

05. Bone Broth

Bone broth is a nourishing and healing drink that's rich in minerals and collagen. It's perfect as a snack or a base for soups and stews.

Ingredients:

2-3 pounds of bones (beef, chicken, or turkey)

1 onion, quartered

2 carrots, chopped

2 celery stalks, chopped

2 tablespoons apple cider vinegar

Sea salt to taste

Water to cover

Instructions:

- ❖ Prepare Bones: If using raw bones, roast them in a 400°F (200°C) oven for 30 minutes to enhance the flavor.

- ❖ Make Broth: Place the bones in a large pot or slow cooker. Add the onion, carrots, celery, apple cider vinegar, and sea salt. Cover with water.

- ❖ Cook: Bring to a boil, then reduce heat and simmer for 12-24 hours. If using a slow cooker, set it to low and cook for the same amount of time.

- ❖ Strain and Store: Strain the broth through a fine mesh sieve to remove the solids. Let it cool, then store in the refrigerator for up to 5 days or freeze for later use.

- ❖ Serve: Enjoy a warm cup of bone broth as a soothing snack or use it as a base for your favorite AIP soups and stews.

These side dishes and snacks are not only compliant with the AIP diet but also packed with flavor and nutrients.

CHAPTER SIX

DESSERTS AND TREATS

Enjoying delicious desserts and treats while following the Autoimmune Paleo (AIP) diet is entirely possible. These recipes are designed to satisfy your sweet tooth without compromising your health goals. Some recommended delightful AIP-friendly desserts that you can easily make at home are listed below;

01. <u>Coconut Macaroons</u>

Coconut macaroons are a simple, yet delicious treat that brings a taste of the tropics to your dessert table. These macaroons are sweet, chewy, and perfect for satisfying your cravings.

<u>Ingredients:</u>

2 cups unsweetened shredded coconut

1/2 cup coconut cream

1/4 cup honey or maple syrup

1 teaspoon vanilla extract

Pinch of sea salt

Instructions:

- ❖ Preheat Oven: Preheat your oven to 325°F (165°C). Line a baking sheet with parchment paper.
- ❖ Mix Ingredients: In a large bowl, combine the shredded coconut, coconut cream, honey, vanilla extract, and sea salt. Mix until well combined.
- ❖ Form Macaroons: Using a tablespoon or a small cookie scoop, form the mixture into small mounds and place them on the prepared baking sheet.
- ❖ Bake: Bake for 20-25 minutes, or until the macaroons are golden brown around the edges.
- ❖ Cool and Serve: Allow the macaroons to cool on the baking sheet for a few minutes before transferring them to a wire rack to cool completely. Enjoy these chewy, coconutty treats.

02. <u>AIP Apple Crisp</u>

AIP apple crisp is a comforting dessert that's perfect for any occasion. This version is made with AIP-compliant ingredients and is just as delicious as the classic.

<u>Ingredients:</u>

4-5 medium apples, peeled, cored, and sliced

2 tablespoons coconut oil

2 tablespoons honey or maple syrup

1 teaspoon cinnamon

1/2 teaspoon ground ginger

1/4 teaspoon sea salt

<u>For the Topping:</u>

1 cup shredded coconut

1/2 cup tigernut flour

1/4 cup coconut oil, melted

2 tablespoons honey or maple syrup

<u>Instructions:</u>

* ❖ Preheat Oven: Preheat your oven to 350°F (175°C). Use coconut oil to coat an 8x8-inch baking dish.

- ❖ Prepare Apples: In a large bowl, toss the apple slices with coconut oil, honey, cinnamon, ground ginger, and sea salt. Spread the apples equally in the baking dish that has been prepared.
- ❖ Make Topping: In a medium bowl, mix together the shredded coconut, tigernut flour, melted coconut oil, and honey until well combined.Distribute the topping generously over the apples.
- ❖ Bake: Bake for 30-35 minutes, or until the apples are tender and the topping is golden brown.
- ❖ Serve the apple crisp when it has cooled for a few minutes. Enjoy warm with a dollop of coconut cream if desired.

0.3 <u>Carob Fudge Bites</u>

These carob fudge bites are rich, chocolaty, and completely AIP-compliant. They're perfect for a quick sweet treat that you can enjoy guilt-free.

Ingredients:

1/2 cup coconut butter

1/4 cup carob powder

2 tablespoons coconut oil

2 tablespoons honey or maple syrup

1 teaspoon vanilla extract

Pinch of sea salt

Instructions:

- ❖ Melt Ingredients: In a small saucepan over low heat, melt the coconut butter, coconut oil, honey, and vanilla extract, stirring constantly until smooth.
- ❖ Mix in Carob: Remove from heat and stir in the carob powder and sea salt until well combined.
- ❖ Chill: Pour the mixture into a silicone mold or a lined baking dish. Refrigerate for at least one hour, or until solid.
- ❖ Cut and Serve: Once set, divide into small bites and savor.
- . Store any leftovers in the refrigerator.

04. <u>Banana Coconut Ice Cream</u>

This banana coconut ice cream is a creamy and refreshing dessert that's perfect for hot days. It's simple to create and only needs a few basic ingredients.

Ingredients:

3 ripe bananas, sliced and frozen

1/2 cup coconut milk

1 teaspoon vanilla extract

2 tablespoons honey (optional)

Instructions:

- ❖ Blend Ingredients: In a high-speed blender or food processor, combine the frozen banana slices, coconut milk, vanilla extract, and honey (if using). Blend until smooth and creamy.
- ❖ Freeze: Transfer the ingredients to a loaf pan or freezer-safe container. Refrigerate for at least two hours or until hard.

❖ Serve: Scoop the ice cream into bowls and enjoy immediately. You can also top it with shredded coconut or fresh fruit for extra flavor.

0.5 Tigernut Flour Cookies

Tigernut flour cookies are a delicious and crunchy treat that's perfect for snacking. These cookies are naturally sweet and have a nutty flavor, making them a delightful addition to your AIP dessert repertoire.

Ingredients:

1 cup tigernut flour

1/4 cup coconut oil, melted

1/4 cup honey or maple syrup

1 teaspoon vanilla extract

1/4 teaspoon sea salt

Instructions:

❖ Preheat Oven: Preheat your oven to 350°F (175°C). Line a baking sheet with parchment paper.

❖ Mix Ingredients: In a large bowl, combine the tigernut flour, melted coconut oil, honey, vanilla extract, and sea salt. Mix until a dough forms.

❖ Form Cookies: Scoop tablespoons of dough onto the prepared baking sheet, flattening them slightly with your fingers or the back of a spoon.

❖ Bake for 10-12 minutes, or till the outsides turn golden brown.

❖ Cool and Serve: Let the cookies cool on the baking sheet for a few minutes before moving them to a wire rack to finish cooling.Enjoy these crunchy, delicious cookies.

These AIP-friendly desserts and treats offer a variety of flavors and textures to satisfy your sweet tooth while supporting your health goals. Enjoy these recipes as part of your journey to better health and well-being.

CHAPTER SEVEN

SAUCES AND CONDIMENTS

Sauces and condiments are essential for adding flavor and excitement to your meals, especially when following the Autoimmune Paleo (AIP) diet. The right sauces can transform simple ingredients into delicious dishes, making your AIP journey more enjoyable. Here are some flavorful and versatile AIP-friendly sauces and condiments you can easily make at home.

01. AIP Mayonnaise

AIP mayonnaise is a creamy and delicious staple that you can use in a variety of dishes, from salads to sandwiches. This version is free from eggs and seed oils, making it perfect for those following the AIP diet.

Ingredients:

1/2 cup coconut butter, melted

1/2 cup extra virgin olive oil

1 tablespoon apple cider vinegar

1 teaspoon Dijon mustard (AIP compliant, if available)

1/2 teaspoon sea salt

1/4 teaspoon garlic powder

1/4 teaspoon onion powder

Instructions:

- ❖ Blend Ingredients: In a high-speed blender or food processor, combine the melted coconut butter, olive oil, apple cider vinegar, Dijon mustard, sea salt, garlic powder, and onion powder.

- ❖ Blend Until Creamy: Blend on high speed until the mixture is smooth and creamy, about 1-2 minutes. You may need to scrape down the sides of the blender to ensure everything is well combined.

- ❖ Store the mayonnaise in a clean container with a cover. Store in the refrigerator for up to a week. The components may separate over time, so stir before use.

02. <u>Coconut Aminos Stir-Fry Sauce</u>

This coconut aminos stir-fry sauce is a fantastic alternative to traditional soy sauce-based stir-fry sauces. It's perfect for adding a savory and slightly sweet flavor to your stir-fried vegetables and proteins.

<u>Ingredients:</u>

1/2 cup coconut aminos

2 tablespoons apple cider vinegar

1 tablespoon honey (optional)

1 garlic clove, minced

1 teaspoon fresh ginger, grated

1/4 teaspoon sea salt

<u>Instructions:</u>

- ❖ Combine Ingredients: In a small bowl, whisk together the coconut aminos, apple cider vinegar, honey (if using), minced garlic, grated ginger, and sea salt.
- ❖ Mix Well: Ensure all the ingredients are well combined.

- ❖ Store: Transfer the sauce to a jar with a lid and store in the refrigerator for up to two weeks.
- ❖ Use: Use this sauce to add flavor to your favorite stir-fried vegetables, meats, and seafood.

03. <u>Avocado Lime Dressing</u>

The avocado lime dressing is creamy, tangy, and full of fresh flavor. It's perfect for drizzling over salads, as a dip for vegetables, or as a sauce for grilled meats.

Ingredients:

1 ripe avocado

1/4 cup extra virgin olive oil

Juice of 1 lime

1 garlic clove, minced

1/4 cup fresh cilantro, chopped

1/2 teaspoon sea salt

1/4 cup water (more as needed)

Instructions:

- ❖ Blend Ingredients: In a blender or food processor, combine the avocado, olive oil, lime juice, minced garlic, chopped cilantro, sea salt, and water.

- ❖ Blend until smooth and creamy. Add extra water as needed to attain the texture you want.

- ❖ Store: Transfer the dressing to a jar with a lid and store in the refrigerator for up to three days.

- ❖ Use: Use this dressing to enhance your salads, as a dip for veggies, or as a sauce for grilled proteins.

04. AIP Barbecue Sauce

This AIP barbecue sauce is tangy and slightly sweet, ideal for coating on grilled meats and vegetables. It is free of nightshades and other major allergies, making it ideal for the AIP diet.

Ingredients:

1/2 cup unsweetened applesauce

1/4 cup coconut aminos

1/4 cup apple cider vinegar

2 tablespoons honey

2 tablespoons molasses

1 teaspoon garlic powder

1 teaspoon onion powder

1/2 teaspoon ground ginger

1/2 teaspoon sea salt

Instructions:

- ❖ Combine Ingredients: In a medium saucepan, combine the applesauce, coconut aminos, apple cider vinegar, honey, molasses, garlic powder, onion powder, ground ginger, and sea salt.
- ❖ Bring the mixture to a boil over medium heat. Lower the heat and let it simmer for 10-15 minutes, stirring periodically, until the sauce thickens.

- ❖ Cool: Remove the sauce from the heat and let it cool.

- ❖ Store: Transfer the barbecue sauce to a jar with a lid and store in the refrigerator for up to one week.

- ❖ Use: Use this barbecue sauce to baste grilled meats, as a dip for roasted vegetables, or as a flavorful marinade.

05. <u>Herb-Infused Olive Oil</u>

Herb-infused olive oil is a simple and versatile condiment that adds a burst of flavor to your dishes. You can use it for drizzling over salads, roasting vegetables, or as a dipping oil for AIP-friendly bread.

<u>Ingredients:</u>

1 cup extra virgin olive oil

2 tablespoons fresh rosemary, chopped

2 tablespoons fresh thyme, chopped

2 garlic cloves, smashed

1 teaspoon lemon zest

Pinch of sea salt

Instructions:

- ❖ Heat Oil: In a small saucepan, heat the olive oil over low heat. Add the chopped rosemary, thyme, smashed garlic, lemon zest, and sea salt.

- ❖ Infuse: Let the mixture simmer on low heat for about 10 minutes, allowing the herbs and garlic to infuse the oil. Be careful not to let the oil get too hot, as it can burn the herbs and garlic.

- ❖ Cool and Strain: Remove the saucepan from the heat and let the oil cool.Sieve the oil through a fine mesh screen to eliminate any herbs or garlic.

- ❖ Store: Transfer the herb-infused olive oil to a clean bottle or jar with a lid. Keep in a cold, dark area for up to a month.

- ❖ Use: Drizzle the herb-infused olive oil over salads, roasted vegetables, or use it as a dipping oil for AIP-friendly bread.

Such AIP-friendly sauces and condiments will enhance the richness and flavor of your meals, making it simpler to adhere to your diet without feeling deprived. Enjoy the diversity and depth that these recipes provide to your cooking skills.

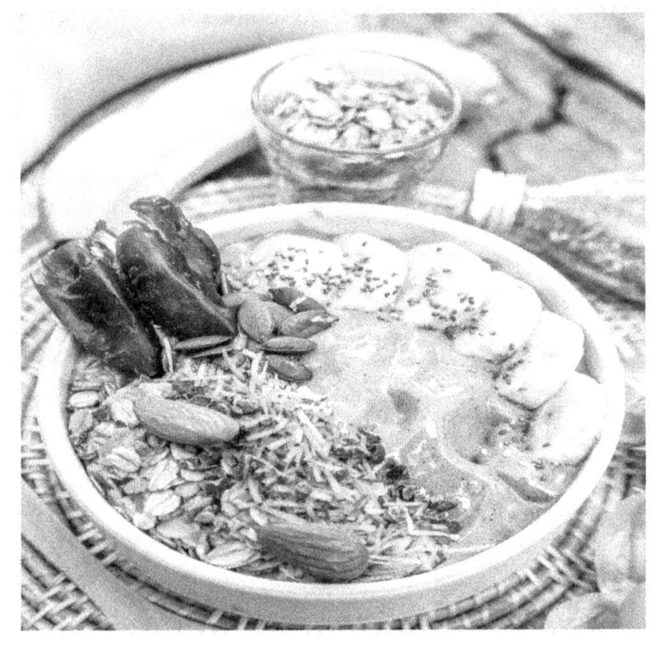

CHAPTER EIGHT

BEVERAGES IN AUTOIMMUNE PALEO DIET

Finding delicious and nourishing beverages can make a big difference when following the Autoimmune Paleo (AIP) diet. These AIP-friendly drinks are designed to support your health while providing refreshing and satisfying options. Here are some tasty beverages that you can enjoy on the AIP diet.

01. Turmeric Ginger Tea

Turmeric ginger tea is a warming, anti-inflammatory beverage that's perfect for soothing your body and mind. This tea is easy to make and packed with healing properties.

Ingredients:

1 cup water

1 teaspoon fresh ginger, grated

1 teaspoon fresh turmeric, grated (or 1/2 teaspoon ground turmeric)

1 tablespoon honey (optional)

Juice of 1/2 lemon

Instructions:

- ❖ Boil Water: Bring the water to a boil in a small saucepan.
- ❖ Add Ginger and Turmeric: Add the grated ginger and turmeric to the boiling water. Lower the heat and allow it simmer for about 10 minutes.
- ❖ Strain: Strain the tea into a cup to remove the ginger and turmeric pieces.
- ❖ Add Honey and Lemon: Stir in the honey (if using) and lemon juice. Adjust sweetness to taste.
- ❖ Serve: Enjoy this soothing and warming tea hot. It's perfect for sipping on a cold day or whenever you need a comforting drink.

02. Coconut Milk Smoothies

Coconut milk smoothies are a creamy and delicious way to enjoy a nutrient-dense beverage. These smoothies can be customized with your favorite AIP-friendly fruits and veggies.

Ingredients:

1 cup coconut milk

1 ripe banana

1/2 cup frozen fruit (strawberries, blueberries, or raspberries)

1/4 cup spinach or kale (optional for extra greens)

1 tablespoon honey (optional)

1/2 teaspoon vanilla extract

Instructions:

❖ Blend Ingredients: In a blender, combine the coconut milk, banana, frozen berries, spinach or kale (if using), honey, and vanilla extract.

❖ Blend at maximum speed until the mixture is smooth and creamy.

- ❖ Pour the smoothie into a glass and drink immediately. This refreshing drink is perfect for breakfast or as a snack.

03. <u>**AIP Bone Broth Elixir**</u>

Bone broth is a powerhouse of nutrients, and turning it into an elixir with added flavors makes it even more enjoyable. This warm, nourishing drink is great for sipping throughout the day.

<u>Ingredients:</u>

1 cup homemade bone broth

1 teaspoon apple cider vinegar

1/4 teaspoon turmeric powder

1/4 teaspoon ground ginger

Pinch of sea salt

1 teaspoon fresh lemon juice

<u>Instructions:</u>

- ❖ Heat Broth: In a small saucepan, heat the bone broth over medium heat until hot but not boiling.

- ❖ Add Ingredients: Stir in the apple cider vinegar, turmeric powder, ground ginger, sea salt, and lemon juice.
- ❖ Mix Well: Whisk the mixture to ensure all the ingredients are well combined.
- ❖ Serve: Pour the elixir into a mug and enjoy it warm.

This nourishing drink is perfect for sipping throughout the day to support your health.

04. <u>Herbal Infusions</u>

Herbal infusions are a gentle and calming way to enjoy the benefits of various herbs. These caffeine-free beverages can be enjoyed hot or cold, depending on your preference.

<u>Ingredients:</u>

1 tablespoon dried chamomile flowers

1 tablespoon dried peppermint leaves

1 tablespoon dried nettle leaves

1 tablespoon dried hibiscus flowers

4 cups boiling water

Instructions:

- ❖ Combine Herbs: In a large teapot or heat proof jar, combine the dried chamomile, peppermint, nettle, and hibiscus.
- ❖ Add Water: Pour the boiling water over the herbs.
- ❖ Steep: Cover and let the herbs steep for 15-20 minutes.
- ❖ Strain: Strain the infusion to remove the herbs.
- ❖ Serve: Enjoy the herbal infusion hot, or let it cool and serve over ice for a refreshing cold drink. Feel free to sweeten with a little honey if desired.

05. Sparkling Fruit Coolers

Sparkling fruit coolers are a fun and refreshing way to enjoy natural flavors without added sugars or artificial ingredients. These drinks are perfect for hot days or when you want something fizzy and fruity.

Ingredients:

1 cup sparkling water

1/2 cup fresh fruit juice (such as watermelon, pineapple, or orange)

1/4 cup fresh fruit (sliced berries, citrus, or melon)

Fresh mint leaves for garnish

Ice cubes

Instructions:

- ❖ Combine Juice and Sparkling Water: In a large glass or pitcher, combine the fresh fruit juice and sparkling water.

- ❖ Add Fruit and Mint: Add the fresh fruit slices and mint leaves.

- ❖ Serve: Fill glasses with ice cubes and pour the sparkling fruit cooler over the ice. Garnish with additional mint leaves if desired. Enjoy this refreshing beverage immediately.

These AIP-friendly beverages provide a variety of flavors and health benefits, making it easier to stay hydrated and satisfied while following the

Autoimmune Paleo diet. Enjoy these drinks as part of your daily routine to support your wellness journey.

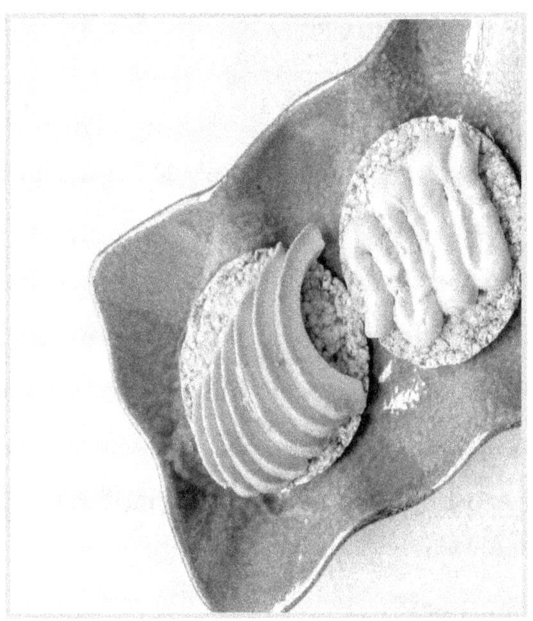

CHAPTER NINE

SPECIAL OCCASIONS AND THE AIP DIET

Special occasions often revolve around food, and it can be challenging to stick to the Autoimmune Paleo (AIP) diet while celebrating holidays, birthdays, picnics, or entertaining guests. However, with a little planning and creativity, you can enjoy delicious and festive meals that align with your dietary needs. Listed below are some suggestions for different special events to make your AIP journey more joyful and fulfilling.

AIP Holiday Feast

Holidays are a time for indulgence and gathering with loved ones, and you don't have to miss out on the festivities because of dietary restrictions. An AIP holiday feast can be just as delicious and comforting as traditional holiday meals.

Main Course: Herb-Roasted Turkey or Chicken

Ingredients:

Whole turkey or chicken, fresh herbs (rosemary, thyme, sage), garlic, lemon, olive oil, sea salt, and black pepper (optional).

Instructions:

- ❖ Preheat the oven to 350°F (175°C).
- ❖ Prepare a mixture of chopped herbs, minced garlic, lemon juice, olive oil, sea salt, and black pepper.
- ❖ Rub this mixture under the skin and on the surface of the bird.
- ❖ Roast according to the weight of the bird, basting occasionally with the juices, until the meat reaches an internal temperature of 165°F (74°C).

Side Dishes:

Roasted Root Vegetables:

- ❖ Mix carrots, parsnips, sweet potatoes, and beets with olive oil, sea salt, and herbs.
- ❖ Roast until tender and caramelized.

AIP Stuffing:

- ❖ Combine cooked ground pork or turkey with diced celery, onions, apples, and fresh herbs.
- ❖ Bake in a dish until golden brown.

Cranberry Sauce:

- ❖ Simmer fresh cranberries with orange juice, a touch of honey, and a pinch of cinnamon until the berries burst and the sauce thickens.

Dessert: AIP Pumpkin Pie

- ❖ Crust: Blend tigernut flour, coconut oil, and a pinch of sea salt to form a dough. Press into a pie dish and bake until golden.
- ❖ Filling: Mix pureed pumpkin, coconut milk, honey, and spices like cinnamon, ginger, and cloves. Pour into the prepared crust and bake until firm.

Birthday Celebration Menu

Birthdays call for celebration, and you can create a festive menu that fits within the AIP guidelines without sacrificing flavor or fun.

Main Course: Grilled Steak with Chimichurri Sauce

Ingredients:

Steak of your choice, olive oil, sea salt, garlic, fresh parsley, fresh cilantro, red wine vinegar, and lemon juice.

Instructions:

- ❖ Season the steak with olive oil and sea salt. Grill to desired doneness.
- ❖ For the chimichurri, blend fresh parsley, cilantro, minced garlic, red wine vinegar, lemon juice, and olive oil. Serve the steak with the chimichurri sauce on top.

<u>Side Dishes:Sweet Potato Fries</u>:

❖ Cut sweet potatoes into fries, toss with olive oil and sea salt, and bake until crispy.

<u>AIP Coleslaw</u>:

❖ Shred cabbage and carrots, and mix with an AIP-friendly mayo dressing (coconut butter, olive oil, apple cider vinegar, and a touch of honey).

<u>Dessert: AIP Birthday Cake</u>

❖ Cake: Blend coconut flour, tapioca flour, honey, coconut oil, and coconut milk. Bake in a round cake pan.

❖ Frosting: Mix coconut cream with a little honey and vanilla extract. Spread on the cooled cake and top with fresh berries.

AIP Picnic Ideas

Picnics are a great way to enjoy the outdoors and a meal with family and friends. The following are some portable and tasty AIP-friendly picnic ideas.

Main Course: AIP Chicken Salad Wraps

Ingredients:

Cooked chicken breast, diced apples, celery, AIP mayo, fresh herbs, large lettuce leaves.

Instructions:

- ❖ Mix diced chicken, apples, celery, and fresh herbs with AIP mayo.
- ❖ Distribute the mixture over broad lettuce leaves and wrap up.

Side Dishes:

Veggie Sticks with Guacamole:

- ❖ Slice cucumbers, carrots, and bell peppers.
- ❖ Serve with homemade guacamole (avocado, lime juice, garlic powder, and sea salt).

Fruit Salad:

- ❖ Mix fresh berries, melon, and citrus segments for a refreshing and sweet side dish.

Dessert: AIP Energy Balls

Ingredients:

Blend dates, shredded coconut, coconut oil, and a pinch of sea salt. Form into tiny balls and chill until hard.

Entertaining Guests with AIP

Hosting a dinner party while on the AIP diet can be a delightful experience for everyone with the right menu that accommodates all dietary needs.

Main Course: Baked Salmon with Lemon and Dill

Salmon fillets, lemon slices, fresh dill, olive oil, sea salt.

Instructions:

- ❖ Preheat the oven to 375°F (190°C).
- ❖ Place salmon fillets on a baking sheet, top with lemon slices, fresh dill, and a drizzle of olive oil.
- ❖ Bake until the salmon is opaque and flakes easily with a fork.

<h1 style="text-align:center"><u>Side Dishes:</u></h1>

AIP Caesar Salad: Romaine lettuce with AIP Caesar dressing (blended olive oil, lemon juice, garlic, anchovy paste, and a touch of honey) and topped with roasted garlic chips.

Roasted Brussels Sprouts: Toss Brussels sprouts with olive oil, sea salt, and garlic powder. Roast until crispy and caramelized.

<h1 style="text-align:center"><u>Dessert:</u></h1>

AIP Coconut Pudding: Coconut milk, honey, gelatin, and vanilla extract.

<h1 style="text-align:center"><u>Instructions:</u></h1>

- ❖ Heat coconut milk and honey in a saucepan until warm.
- ❖ Sprinkle in gelatin and stir until dissolved.
- ❖ Add vanilla extract, pour into serving cups, and chill until set.

Traveling and Eating Out on AIP

Traveling and dining out can be challenging on the AIP diet, but with some preparation and flexibility, you can maintain your dietary needs without stress.

Tips for Traveling:

Pack Snacks: Bring AIP-friendly snacks like beef jerky, dried fruit, raw veggies, and AIP energy bars.

Stay Hydrated: Carry a water bottle and herbal teas to stay hydrated and avoid the temptation of sugary drinks.

Research Restaurants: Look up restaurant menus in advance to find AIP-friendly options or places willing to accommodate dietary restrictions.

Tips for Eating Out:

Communicate with the Staff: Don't hesitate to inform the restaurant staff about your dietary needs. Most places are happy to accommodate.

Simple Choices: Opt for simple dishes like grilled meats, steamed vegetables, and fresh salads.

Request dressings and sauces on the side to prevent unknown ingredients

Custom Orders: Feel free to customize your order. Most restaurants can prepare dishes without certain ingredients if you ask politely.

With planning ahead of time and becoming creative with your meals, you can enjoy special occasions, travel, and dining out while adhering to the AIP diet. These suggestions will allow you to appreciate and cherish each moment without jeopardizing your health and well-being.

CHAPTER TEN

REINTRODUCTIONS AND MAINTENANCE IN AIP DIET

The Autoimmune Paleo (AIP) diet is a powerful tool for managing autoimmune conditions by eliminating foods that can trigger inflammation and immune responses. However, the AIP diet isn't meant to be a permanent restriction. Once you've given your body time to heal, you can start reintroducing foods. This process, known as reintroduction, is critical for identifying specific food sensitivities and customizing your long-term diet to best support your health.

When and How to Reintroduce Foods

Reintroduction should only begin after you've experienced a significant reduction in symptoms and have maintained this improvement for at least 30 days. This period allows your body to heal from the inflammation caused by trigger foods and provides a clearer baseline for identifying reactions when foods are reintroduced.

Steps for Reintroduction:

Choose the Right Time: Ensure you're in a stable environment without major stressors, travel, or illness. Your body needs to be in a calm state to accurately assess reactions.

Introduce Foods One at a Time: Reintroduce one food every 3-7 days. This slow approach helps you accurately identify any reactions to each food.

Start with the Least Allergenic Foods: Begin with foods that are less likely to cause reactions, such as egg yolks, seed spices, and ghee. Avoid high-risk foods like grains and dairy initially.

Eat a Small Amount: Start with a small amount of the food, like a teaspoon of ghee or a bite of egg yolk, and wait 15 minutes. If you have no reaction, gradually increase the amount over the next 24 hours.

Monitor for Reactions: Watch for symptoms such as digestive issues, headaches, skin changes, joint pain, fatigue, or mood changes. Record any reactions in a food journal.

Assess and Decide: If you experience no negative reactions, include the food into your diet in moderation. If you do have a reaction, remove the food and wait until symptoms subside before trying another.

Tracking Symptoms and Progress

Keeping a detailed journal is essential during the reintroduction phase. Documenting what you eat and any symptoms that arise helps you make clear connections between foods and your body's responses.

What to Track:

Food Intake: Note the food introduced, the amount, and the time consumed.

Symptoms: Record any physical, emotional, or cognitive symptoms. Be specific about the type, intensity, and duration of symptoms.

Overall Health: Track your sleep, stress levels, exercise, and other lifestyle factors that could influence your health.

Progress: Regularly review your journal to identify patterns and trends. This review can help you make informed decisions about your diet.

Tips for Long-Term Success

Transitioning from the elimination phase of the AIP diet to a sustainable, personalized diet requires patience and careful planning. These are some strategies for long-term success:

Maintain flexibility: Your nutritional needs may change as time goes on.

Be willing to adjust your diet as your body heals and your tolerance for certain foods improves or changes.

Focus on Nutrient Density: Continue to prioritize nutrient-dense foods such as vegetables, fruits, lean proteins, and healthy fats. These foods promote overall health and immunological function.

Listen to your body. Pay close attention to how your body reacts to various meals and modify your diet accordingly. If a food that was previously tolerated starts causing issues, consider removing it again.

Manage Stress: Stress can exacerbate autoimmune symptoms. Adopt stress-reduction strategies like mindfulness, meditation, yoga, and deep breathing exercises into your daily routine.

Maintain a Support System: Connect with others who understand the challenges of managing an autoimmune condition. Support groups, online communities, or a nutritionist specializing in AIP can provide valuable guidance and encouragement.

Prepare for Social Situations: Social events and dining out might be difficult. Plan ahead by checking restaurant menus, bringing AIP-friendly dishes to potlucks, or eating before you go out to avoid temptation.

Personalizing Your AIP Diet

The ultimate goal of the AIP diet is to create a personalized eating plan that supports your health and well-being. This personalized approach ensures you get the nutrients you need while avoiding foods that trigger your symptoms.

Steps to Personalization:

Identify Safe Foods: Through the reintroduction process, determine which foods your body tolerates well. These become the staples of your diet.

Eliminate Trigger Foods: Identify and eliminate foods that cause adverse reactions. These may be permanently excluded or re-evaluated periodically.

Diversify Your Diet: Include a wide variety of foods within your safe list to ensure you get a broad spectrum of nutrients. Try with new recipes and cooking techniques to keep your dinners exciting.

Balance Macronutrients: Ensure your diet includes a balance of proteins, fats, and carbohydrates tailored to your body's needs. Adjust portions based on your activity level, metabolism, and health goals.

Supplement Wisely: Consider supplements if you have nutrient deficiencies that cannot be met through diet alone. Consult a healthcare provider for guidance on which supplements are essential.

Monitor and Adjust: Regularly assess your health and adjust your diet as needed. Life changes, stress levels, and health conditions can all impact your dietary needs.

Reintroductions and maintenance on the AIP diet require a mindful and systematic approach, but the benefits of understanding your body and managing your health are worth the effort. With careful planning and patience, you can enjoy a varied and satisfying diet that supports your long-term health and well-being.

RESOURCES IN AIP DIET

Taking on the Autoimmune Paleo (AIP) diet can be stressful., but having the right resources can make the journey smoother and more enjoyable. Even if you're seeking ingredient substitutes. shopping lists, cooking tools, or support networks, tThis guide will help you explore the AIP diet with ease.

AIP Ingredient Substitutions

One of the biggest challenges of the AIP diet is figuring out how to replace common ingredients that are off-limits. Listed are some handy substitutions to keep your recipes compliant and delicious.

Grains and Flours:

Almond Flour: Use tigernut flour or coconut flour as a substitute. Bear in mind that coconut flour is quite absorbent, so use little of it.

Cornstarch: Arrowroot powder or tapioca starch works well as a thickener in sauces and soups.

Dairy:

Milk: Coconut milk or tigernut milk can replace cow's milk in most recipes.

Butter: Use coconut oil or lard for baking and cooking.

Cheese: Nutritional yeast can provide a cheesy flavor without the dairy.

Eggs:

Eggs in Baking: Use gelatin eggs (1 tablespoon gelatin mixed with 3 tablespoons water) or a blend of mashed banana and baking soda for binding in recipes.

Legumes:

Peanut Butter: Substitute with sunflower seed butter or tigernut butter.

Soy Sauce: Coconut aminos provide a similar umami flavor without the soy.

Nightshades:

Tomatoes: Replace with a blend of cooked carrots and beets for a similar color and slight sweetness.

Potatoes: Sweet potatoes, yams, or plantains are great alternatives.

AIP Shopping List

Having a well-organized shopping list can simplify your grocery trips and ensure you have everything you need for your AIP meals. Here's a basic AIP shopping list to get you started.

Proteins

Grass-fed beef

Pastured chicken and turkey

Wild-caught fish and seafood

Organ meats (liver, heart)

Pork

Vegetables:

Leafy greens (kale, spinach, collard greens)

Cruciferous vegetables (broccoli, cauliflower, Brussels sprouts)

Root vegetables (sweet potatoes, carrots, beets)

Squash (butternut, acorn, spaghetti)

Fresh herbs (parsley, cilantro, basil)

Fruits:

Berries (blueberries, strawberries, raspberries)

Apples

Pears

Bananas

Citrus fruits (oranges, lemons, limes)

Fats:

Coconut oil

Olive oil

Avocado oil

Lard or tallow

Avocados

Pantry Staples:

Coconut aminos

Apple cider vinegar

Coconut milk

Bone broth

Sea salt

Gelatin

Snacks:

Dried fruit (without added sugar)

Coconut flakes

Plantain chips

AIP-friendly jerky

Tigernuts

Useful Tools and Equipment for AIP Cooking

Having the right kitchen tools can make AIP cooking more efficient and enjoyable. Here are some essential items:

Basic Tools:

Sharp Knives: Essential for chopping vegetables and preparing meats.

Cutting Boards: Have separate boards for vegetables and meats to avoid cross-contamination.

Measuring Cups and Spoons: For accurate measurements in recipes.

Mixing Bowls: Various sizes for mixing ingredients.

Cooking Equipment:

High-Quality Blender: For smoothies, soups, and sauces.

Food Processor: Great for making AIP flours, chopping vegetables, and blending ingredients.

Instant Pot or Slow Cooker: Perfect for making bone broth, soups, and stews with ease.

Cast Iron Skillet: Versatile and ideal for cooking meats and vegetables.

Baking Sheets and Pans: For roasting vegetables and baking AIP treats.

Spiralizer: To make zucchini noodles and other vegetable-based pasta substitutes.

Recommended Reading and Websites

Support and Community Resources

Having a supportive community can make a huge difference when following the AIP diet. Connecting with others who understand your challenges can provide encouragement and practical advice.

Online Communities:

Facebook Groups: Search for AIP-specific groups where members share recipes, tips, and support.

Reddit (r/AutoImmunePaleo): A community where you can ask questions, share experiences, and find inspiration.

Instagram: Follow AIP bloggers and influencers for daily meal ideas and motivation.

Local Support:

Meetup.com: Look for local AIP or paleo groups that organize meetups and events.

Health Practitioners: Seek out nutritionists or dietitians who specialize in the AIP diet and can provide personalized guidance.

Cooking Classes: Find AIP-friendly cooking classes in your area to learn new skills and recipes.

Coaching and Mentorship:

Certified AIP Coaches: These professionals offer personalized support and guidance to help you move around the AIP diet. They can provide meal plans, troubleshooting advice, and emotional support.

Consultations: Many AIP experts offer one-on-one consultations to help you tailor the diet to your specific needs and goals.

With these resources, you'll be well-equipped to manage your AIP diet successfully. Remember, the journey is unique for everyone, so take the time to find what works best for you and reach out for support when needed. Your health and well-being are worth the effort.

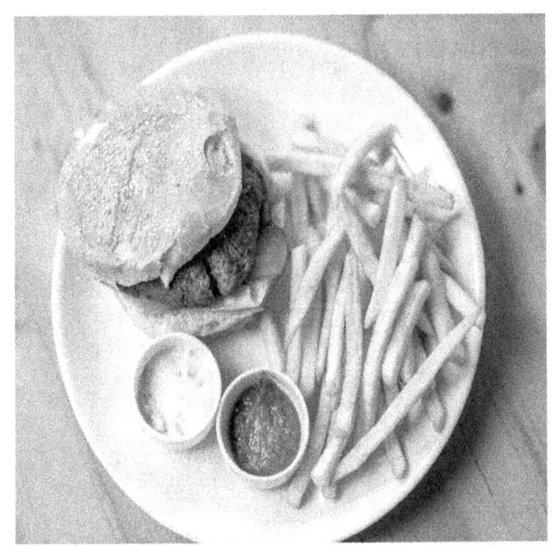

CONCLUSION

Starting the Autoimmune Paleo (AIP) diet is a transformative journey that demands commitment, patience, and an open mind. This cookbook is intended to be your partner on your journey, providing not only recipes but also advice, inspiration, and encouragement.

Appreciate the Journey

The AIP diet is more than simply a style of eating; it's a comprehensive approach to wellness. Focusing on nutrient-dense, anti-inflammatory meals gives your body the best opportunity of recuperating and thriving. The path may be difficult—whether it's managing social situations, finding adequate substitutes for your favorite foods, or simply keeping motivated—but remember that each step you take is a step toward better health and well-being.

Celebrating Small Wins

As you've seen throughout this cookbook, there's no shortage of delicious and satisfying meals that fit within the AIP framework. From hearty breakfasts and nourishing lunches to comforting dinners and delightful desserts, you can enjoy a wide variety of foods that support your health goals. Celebrate each small win along the way—whether it's successfully reintroducing a food, discovering a new favorite recipe, or simply feeling better in your day-to-day life.

Finding Your Balance

One of the most empowering aspects of the AIP diet is learning to listen to your body and personalize your approach. What works for one individual may not work for another, and that's fine. Use the reintroduction phase to identify which foods work for you and which don't. This personalized approach will help you create a sustainable diet that fits your unique needs and lifestyle.

Building a Support System

You do not have to go through this path alone. Connect with others who understand the challenges and triumphs of managing an autoimmune condition. Whether through online communities, local support groups, or working with AIP-certified coaches, having a support system can provide encouragement, practical advice, and a sense of camaraderie.

Looking Forward

The AIP diet is not just about restriction; it's about discovery. You'll discover new foods, new recipes, and new ways of taking care of yourself. You'll also discover resilience and strength within yourself as you go through this path to better health.

As you continue on your AIP journey, remember to be kind to yourself. There will be ups and downs, but every effort you make is a testament to your commitment to your health. Keep experimenting, keep learning, and keep moving forward.

Thank you for allowing this cookbook to be a part of your journey. May it serve as a source of nourishment, inspiration, and support as you adopt the AIP lifestyle. Here's to your health, happiness, and the many delicious meals ahead.

www.ingramcontent.com/pod-product-compliance
Lightning Source LLC
Chambersburg PA
CBHW070740250726
48662CB00004B/1598